Contents

1 **Why Mindfulness? Stress in the Healthcare Workplace**

Impact of Stress on Health and Well-being   1

   Signs of Stress   2

The Mind–Body Connection   3

   Examples of Mind–Body Therapies   3

4 **Integrating Mindfulness into Nursing Practice**

   Qualities of Mindfulness and Their Implications for Nursing Practice   6

The Science of Mindfulness   7

   A Mindfulness Experience   8

Mindfulness and Patient Safety   9

Mindfulness Practices   9

   Developing Your Mind–Body Connection   10

Starting a Meditation Practice   12

STOP: Moving Out of Autopilot   12

Relational Mindfulness   13

Bringing Mindfulness into the Workplace   13

The Path to Mindfulness   13

   A Guide for Your Mindfulness Journey   14

15 **References**

18 **Suggested Readings and Resources**

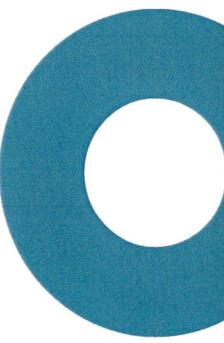

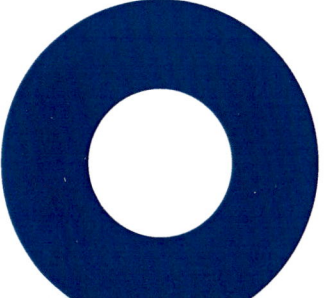

Why Mindfulness?
Stress in the Healthcare Workplace

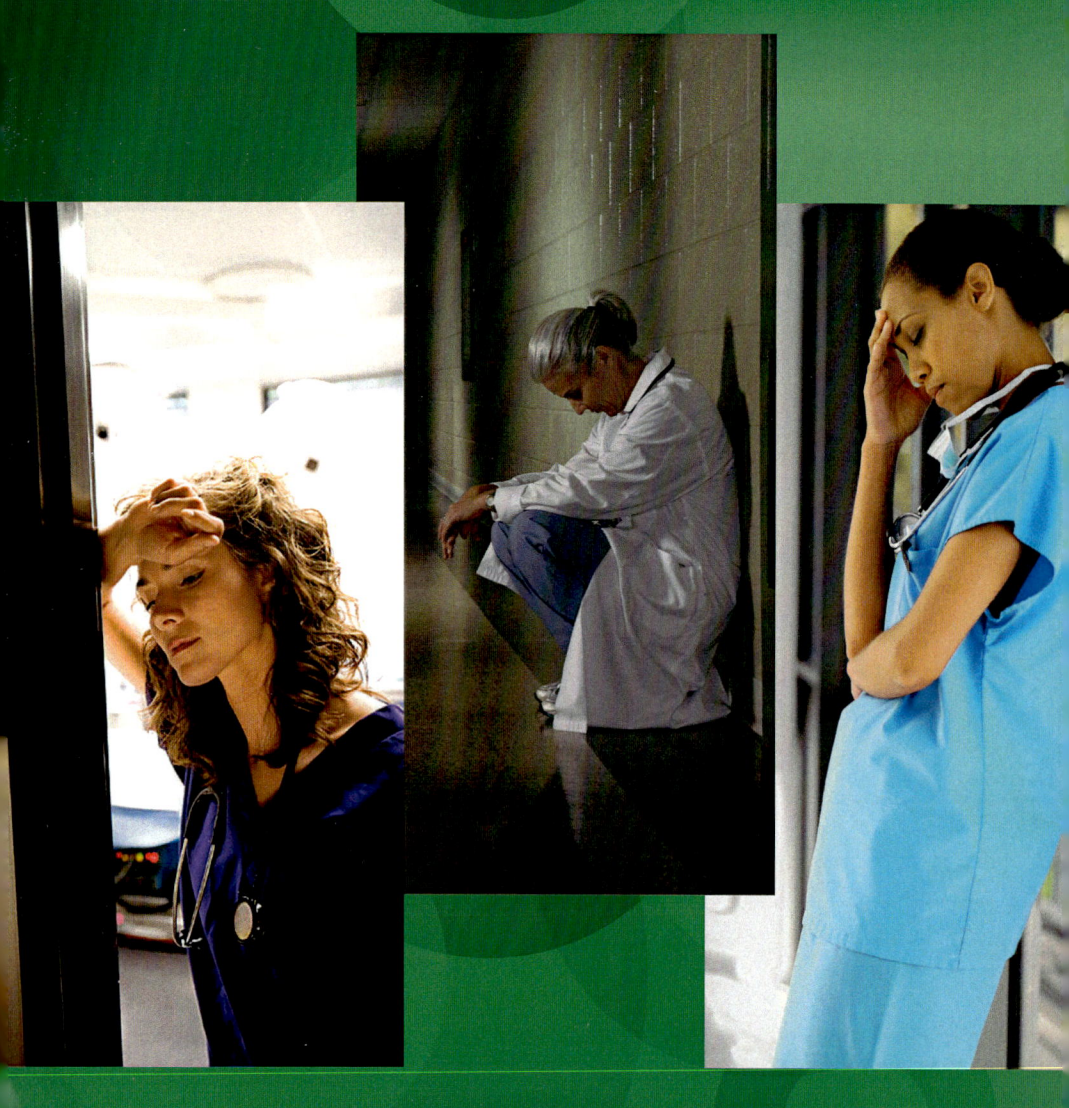

The rapidly changing healthcare landscape presents nurses with a number of challenges to providing safe, affordable, and high quality care. Nurses are being called upon more than ever to serve in expanded roles, deliver primary care and preventive services, provide care coordination, and educate patients and their families about the importance of taking personal accountability for their health and healthcare choices. As nurses, we often find ourselves in work environments with fewer financial resources, poor communication practices, and minimal support systems. These unhealthy work environments can lead to a number of negative outcomes including burnout, low job satisfaction, high turnover, and high degrees of stress (Gilboa, Shirom, Fried, & Cooper, 2008; Zangaro & Soeken, 2007). Evidence also strongly suggests that our unmanaged stress can have detrimental effects on patient care and safety (Aiken, Clarke, Sloane, Sochalski, & Silber, 2002; Elfering, Semmer, & Grebner, 2006; Jennings, 2008). The rapid rate of new technologies in the workplace and the plethora of information to be processed contributes to the feeling that life is increasingly complex and frenetic; it pushes us into the throes of living life as "human doings" versus "human beings." Not surprisingly, nurses often care for others at the expense of themselves.

In light of the shortage of resources, the constantly changing healthcare environment, the demands of an aging, a more complex population, and the millions of people receiving coverage for the first time (America's Health Insurance Plans, 2013), it is critical that we find ways to support ourselves in order to remain actively engaged and employed in nursing while providing safe, compassionate, and patient-centered care. We need new tools and resources to build resilience and address known and unknown challenges that we encounter on a daily basis. The health of families, communities, and the U.S. population as a whole heavily depends upon our positive influence. Effectively caring for others begins first with caring for ourselves.

The practice of mindfulness is one way nurses can care for themselves. Mindfulness has been described as present-centered awareness, or being fully present in the moment and being nonjudgmental. Shapiro and colleagues (2006) note that mindfulness is a moment-by-moment process that involves the interwoven components of intention (purpose), attention (observing), and attitude (how we attend), and Brown and Ryan (2003, p. 823) describe mindfulness as being "characterized by clarity and vividness of current experience and functioning." Cultivation of this state of attention to present moment experiences can be achieved through a number of contemplative practices such as meditation and yoga, or even through engaging in creative processes or spending time in nature. As one learns mindfulness techniques, this stance of open curiosity and acceptance can be applied in basic everyday moments as well as during times of increased pressure, stress, or emotional upheaval.

Impact of Stress on Health and Well-being

Mindfulness can be particularly helpful in dealing with the ups and downs of life by altering how we experience even challenging events. Stress is an inevitable part of life and the human condition. We all live with a number of uncertainties, challenges, pain, and suffering. We simply cannot control all of the events of our lives. Individual stress responses are highly variable and many can be maladaptive, resulting in estrangement or isolation from the beautiful simplicities of life and disconnectedness from ourselves and others.

Signs of Stress

Physical signs:
- Headaches
- Back/neck pain
- Nausea/upset stomach
- High blood pressure/palpitations
- Fatigue/low energy
- Insomnia
- Frequent colds/infections

Psychological signs:
- Anxiety
- Depression
- Irritability
- Lack of focus/concentration
- Forgetfulness
- Disengagement
- Feeling overwhelmed

As healthcare workers, we can often feel overwhelmed with our roles as care providers and leaders of other nurses. Mindfulness helps us to learn more about ourselves and how we relate to our world; in essence, changing our relationship with life (Smalley & Winston, 2010). Surveys and research identify stress and unhealthy work environments as significant sources of concern of negative impacts on personal health and professional satisfaction (American Nurses Association [ANA], 2011; Buerhaus, Donelan, Ulrich, Norman, & Dittus, 2006; Jennings, 2008).

Simply put, stress occurs when we experience a real or perceived threat which sets in motion a series of responses as our bodies attempt to maintain homeostasis. Hormones are released, most notably epinephrine and cortisol, to prepare for the extra energy needed to respond to real or imagined events (O'Connor, O'Halloran, & Shanahan, 2000). From an evolutionary perspective, this acute stress response used to serve us well by protecting us from real physical threats. However, because most of the stressors found in modern life are chronic in nature, they continually impede proper regulation of the two parts of the autonomic nervous system: sympathetic (fight or flight) and parasympathetic (rest and restoration). While the fight or flight response may assure survival in the short term, it has deleterious effects on every system of the body after it becomes chronic and overwhelming because individuals are unable to engage in the important relaxation response (Benson, 1975).

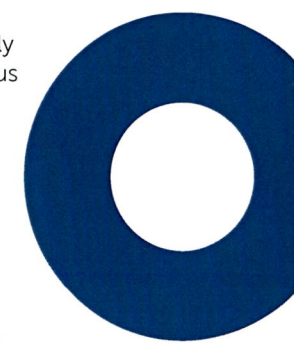

The Mind—Body Connection

An intricate relationship exists between the mind, emotions, and the physical processes of the body. Thoughts and thought habits can positively or negatively affect our physical well-being. Similarly, the choices we make regarding our physical bodies, such as diet, exercise, and rest, among other things, can also positively or negatively affect our mental states. The mind and body are inseparable; they share a common chemical language that constantly communicates back and forth (Hart, 2008).

Fortunately, there are a number of practices that we can utilize to enhance the mind's positive impact on the body as well as the body's positive impact on the mind. These self-care practices have been shown to increase awareness of mental states, regulate emotions, and enhance overall health and well-being.

Examples of Mind—Body Therapies

- Relaxation techniques
- Massage therapy
- Yoga
- Acupuncture
- Meditation
- Tai chi
- Qigong (chi gong)
- Biofeedback
- Guided imagery
- Creative therapies

Integrating Mindfulness into Nursing Practice

The future hasn't happened yet and the past is gone. So I think the only moment we have is right here and now, and I try to make the best of those moments, the moments that I'm in.
—Annie Lennox

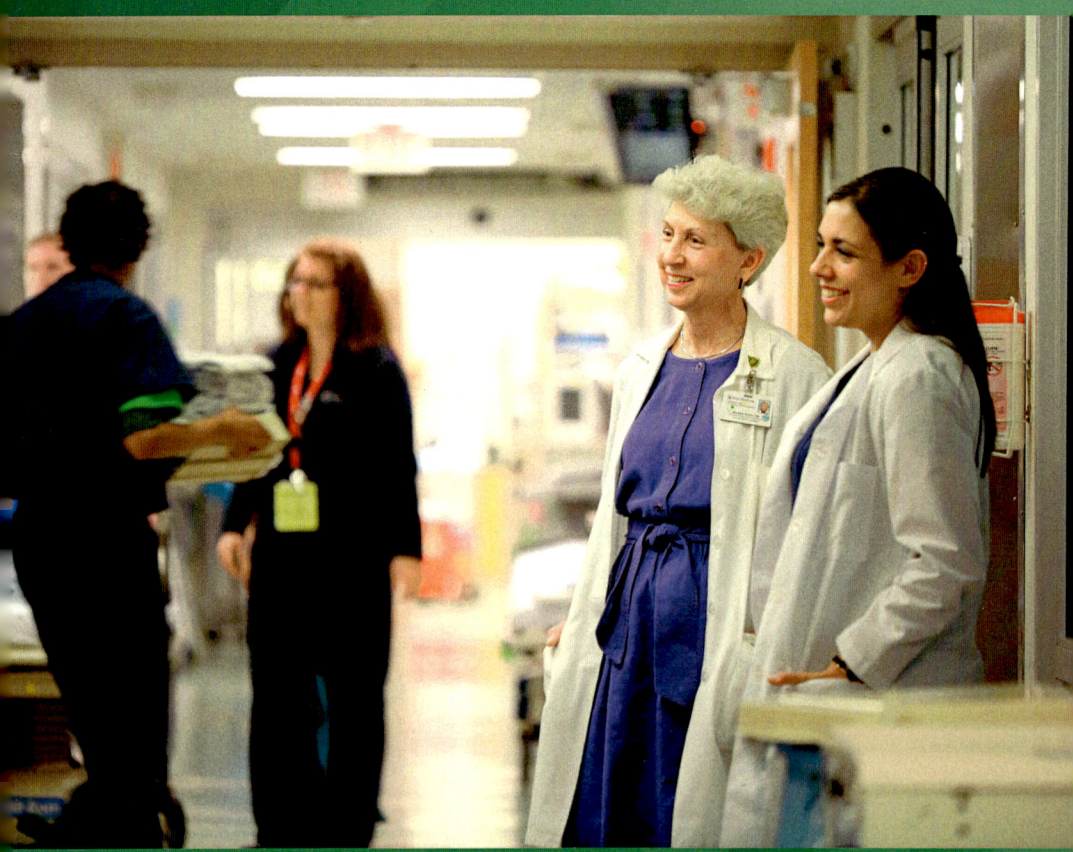

One of the most powerful tools for enhancing self-care is the practice of mindfulness. Just as mindfulness can be helpful for achieving and sustaining a balanced state of mind and emotional state in our day-to-day lives, mindfulness can also be very helpful when dealing with physical or emotional pain, enhancing focus and attention, boosting creativity, potentiating performance including safe care practices, potentiating the therapeutic relationship, and enhancing compassion and empathy for self and others—all crucial for those in the caring profession. Mindfulness, an ancient practice of cultivating the ability to be fully present in each moment in openness and acceptance, is gaining the attention of the healthcare community and the public in general. Many people show great interest in bringing mindfulness into all aspects of daily life, including exploring ways to prevent illness, improve well-being, enhance performance, and alleviate pain and suffering.

While rooted in Buddhist tradition dating back more than 2,500 years, the secular introduction of mindfulness into health care can be attributed to Jon Kabat-Zinn at the University of Massachusetts. In 1979, Kabat-Zinn first offered a group-based program called Mindfulness Based Stress Reduction (MBSR) to a complex clinical population as a complement to traditional medical treatment (Kabat-Zinn, 2009).

In his seminal work, *Full Catastrophe Living: Using the Wisdom of Your Body and the Mind to Face Stress, Pain, and Illness,* Jon Kabat-Zinn (2009) describes seven attitudinal factors that constitute the major pillars of mindfulness practice: non-judging, patience, a beginner's mind, trust, non-striving, acceptance, and letting go. Each of these qualities of mindfulness and their potential application to nursing practice to deliver safer, higher quality, more patient-centered care are described in Table 1.

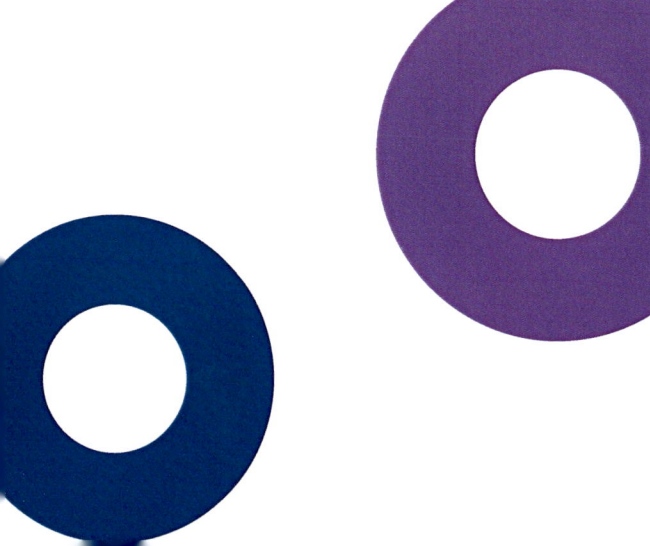

Table 1. Qualities of Mindfulness and Their Implications for Nursing Practice

Mindfulness Quality	Application to Nursing Practice
Non-judging	Becoming more aware of the prevalent habit of categorizing people and events as good, bad, or indifferent.
Patience	Gaining the wisdom to know and accept the fact that some things must unfold in their own time.
Beginner's Mind (Openness)	Seeing things as if for the first time, allowing oneself to be receptive to all possibilities.
Trust	Trusting in one's own wisdom, enabling the cultivation of trust in others.
Non-striving	Enhancing the ability to deeply experience the present without the tension of goal or achievement orientation.
Acceptance	Seeing things as they actually are rather than how one wishes them to be.
Letting Go (Non-attachment)	Allowing thoughts, feelings, and experiences to come and go without getting entangled.

Now, after more than 30 years of research, we know participation in mindfulness practices can improve the physical and mental health and the quality of life of diverse clinical and nonclinical populations. Mindfulness has been shown to increase empathy, compassion, and serenity and to enhance both care provider and patient experience (Krasner et al., 2009; Sansoucie et al., 2006; Shapiro, Astin, Bishop, & Cordova, 2005).

Mindfulness, according to Kabat-Zinn (2009), is purposefully paying attention in the present moment, with a stance of acceptance and non-judgment. By definition, mindful awareness—mindfulness—means being awake and aware, even aware of one's awareness. Contrasting awareness is the notion of operating on "autopilot" by being lost in thoughts of the past or the future (Smalley & Winston, 2010). Only when we operate with awareness are we able to access our deeper resources and remain present to our moment-by-moment experiences. By learning to focus our attention through directing and shaping the mind, we can wake up from mindlessness and living life on autopilot (Siegel, 2007).

While the practices of cultivating mindfulness can be simple to implement, they do require regular practice to reap the benefits. The practice is actually quite simple, yet we test the default mode of the mind, which is to wander. The default state of the human mind is distraction. Thus, mindfulness practice requires discipline and a strong intention to overcome tendencies toward distraction and mindlessness.

As nurses, we are optimally positioned to initiate a personal mindfulness practice to enhance our own health and well-being as well as teach patients how to use these techniques to lower stress and improve their health and wellness.

The Science of Mindfulness

Studies show that participation in mindfulness practices leads to a wide range of physical, emotional, and behavioral changes. The practice of stabilizing the mind and cultivating a state of calm allows us to observe our surroundings with an enhanced ability to respond versus to react reflexively. By attending to the present in our minds and in our bodies at any given moment, we can make wiser choices, thereby choosing a path that does less harm to self and others. Mindfulness helps us look at real or perceived threats in a more objective manner and can be useful at every stage of the emotional process (Rosenberg, 2013).

Mindfulness meditation has been demonstrated to reduce the frequency and intensity of chronic pain, lower anxiety, improve mood disturbances associated with depression, and to improve the duration and quality of sleep (Grossman, Niemann, Schmidt, & Walach, 2004; McCarney, Schulz, & Grey, 2012). By engaging the relaxation response, and lowering stress and the harmful effects of chronic stress, mindfulness helps to lower inflammation and boost the immune response— both of which are compromised in the face of prolonged stress (Davidson et al., 2003).

Evidence shows that when attention is focused on the present moment, individuals are happier and report lower levels of anxiety and an increased sense of well-being (Greeson, 2009; Killingsworth & Gilbert, 2010; Zeidan et al., 2013). This same ability to focus on the present may also predict longevity. The length of telomeres, the DNA-based caps that protect the ends of the chromosomes, typically shorten with age or severe stress, which provides an early indication of disease and mortality (Lin, Epel, & Blackburn, 2011). Scientists have explored whether a tendency toward mind wandering is associated with this telomere length. After adjusting for stress levels, there appears to be some association between the length of telomeres and the degree of mind wandering; less mind wandering is suggestive of a more favorable cellular milieu and increased telomere length (Epel et al., 2013).

Mindfulness training has been shown to enhance working memory and test-taking performance in high school students. A two-week mindfulness training program was found to lower mind wandering and improve GRE scores in the areas of reading comprehension and working memory capacity (Mrazek, Franklin, Phillips, Baird, & Schooler, 2013). Similarly, researchers testing mindfulness with the military found that offering a brief mindfulness training program during the high-stress pre-deployment period resulted in higher levels of working memory capacity and positive affect, particularly for those military personnel engaged in mindfulness practice (Jha, Stanley, Kiyonaga, Wong, & Gelfand, 2010).

Some of the most powerful benefits of mindfulness relate to changes in the function and structure of the brain. The brain has the ability to form new neural connections throughout our lives (neuroplasticity), and practices such as mindful meditation can lead to these changes (Hölzel et al, 2011). Following even short-term mindfulness programs, the fight or flight part of the brain, called the amygdala, becomes smaller while the parts of the brain associated with working memory, attention, and emotional integration (cerebral cortex) become thicker

(Hölzel et al., 2011). In healthcare workers, mindfulness training and practice has led to a variety of positive outcomes: stress reduction, lower levels of personal and professional burnout, increased compassion for self and others, a cultivation of empathy and serenity, and generally enhanced physical and psychological health and well-being of those caring for others (Bazarko, Cate, Azocar & Kreitzer, 2013).

With so many possibilities to improve the lives of clinical and non-clinical populations, mindfulness can be thought of as a foundation for overall health and well-being—a crucial element for achieving the highest quality of life possible. Thankfully, this is a self-care practice that is accessible to all.

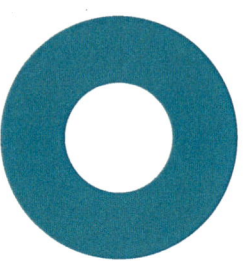

A Mindfulness Experience

- If you wish, find a moment when you can attend to your present moment in terms of the physical, emotional, and thinking self.
- As best you can, bring your awareness first to your thoughts and explore the nature of your thoughts.
    - What are you aware of in your mind?
    - What is the nature of your thinking and what thoughts are you encountering right now?
    - Is your thinking clear? Is it foggy?
    - Are your thoughts recollecting things from the past or planning for the future? Are your thoughts related to your present reality?
    - Just notice what is present, without judging or trying to change anything in your experience.
- Now, bring your attention to your emotions, to your heart center.
    - How would you describe your mood or emotional tone?
    - Do you find anxiety, fear, peacefulness, or anything else?
    - Again, just notice what is present for you with open receptivity and curiosity.
- Finally, bring your attention to the sensations of the physical body.
    - Notice what you are aware of in your body.
    - Do you notice tension, fatigue, high or low energy, calm or ease?
    - What do you notice about the quality of your natural breathing? Breathing is a process; the intent here is to be aware of a breath at a time.

Mindfulness and Patient Safety

Patient safety is of considerable interest to both providers and recipients of health care. The complexities of our healthcare environment present many challenges for nurses and other healthcare workers in delivering safe, patient-centered, and high quality care. Mindfulness can play a key role in creating a culture of safety and enhancing individual clinician performance. Many errors in health care derive from cognitive biases or fixed mental models; these errors include a tendency to make decisions and/or take action with limited information or limited processing of available information, acting in self-interest, demonstrating overconfidence, or showing attachment to previous experiences (Baron, 2007; Croskerry, 2003). By cultivating metacognition, or the ability to become more aware of one's thoughts and thinking processes, an individual may enhance their decision-making skills. Mindfulness can also be seen as an effective de-biasing strategy leading both to greater awareness of one's own experiences, including thinking, emotions, and bodily sensations, and to a nonjudgmental awareness of the present moment (Sibinga & Wu, 2010).

Bringing these qualities of mindfulness into nursing practice could improve patient safety by mitigating the effects of healthcare providers' cognitive biases. And, of course, what is good for the patient is also good for the nurse. The benefits of mindfulness may also accrue to our own well-being: lowering our stress, enhancing compassion for self and others, increasing empathy, and reducing burnout, which all lead to greater job satisfaction.

Mindfulness Practices

Typical components of mindfulness practices include mindful meditation, mindful movement in the form of yoga and walking meditation, and other techniques aimed at cultivating the ability to attend to the present moment, calm the mind and body, and engage the relaxation response. To best understand mindfulness, it is helpful to experience it first-hand. If you would like, you are invited to participate in a mindfulness experience (described briefly in the sidebar on the previous page and in more detail on the next), in order to understand the practice.

During mindfulness practices, we learn to focus our attention on a neutral object, often the sensation of breath in the body. By doing so, we can cultivate the ability to increase our concentration and focus on the present moment rather than worrying about the past or planning for future events.

Typical mindfulness programs teach participants how to repeatedly focus attention on present moment awareness with acceptance and emotional non-reactivity. The nature of the human mind is to wander; this is, in fact, the default mode of the brain. While highly variable by individual and task, it is estimated that we spend almost 50 per cent of our time thinking about something other than what we are doing in the present moment (Killingsworth & Gilbert, 2010).

• 9

Developing Your Mind–Body Connection

- Begin the practice by assuming a seated position on a chair or a cushion. Maintain an upright, alert, yet relaxed posture. You may keep your eyes open or closed, depending upon your comfort level and degree of sleepiness. Be sure to turn off any technology that might interrupt your practice.
- Start by bringing some gratitude to yourself for taking the time for self-care, knowing that this is an act of self-love. If you would like, take a couple deep breaths in and out, inviting relaxation and ease into your day, as best you can.
- Become aware of your body sitting here. Notice sensations in the body: the weight of the body, your feet touching the floor or your legs against the chair or cushion. Feel the whole body sitting here.
- Simply notice and acknowledge what is present and just let it be. There is no need to judge or change anything. When sensing the body, you may notice areas of tightness or tension; try to soften and relax those areas if that works for you; if not, just let it be.
- As you notice sensations of the body, you may notice sensations of the breath, the natural breath. Breathe normally as you always do when you are not paying attention.
- As you breathe in, be aware of breathing in; as you breathe out, be aware that you are breathing out. In this practice, the breath is our anchor; it is the object of our attention. The place we can always come back to whether in the busyness of the day or during quiet moments.
- Now bring your attention to where you feel the breath most strongly. It could be in the rising and falling of the abdomen, or the chest, or the bit of turbulence at the nostrils when air comes in and out of the nose. Just pick one place that is most vivid to you, noticing the full cycle of the breath. Explore with curiosity the entire cycle of the in breath, the fast turn, and the entire cycle of the out breath, the fast turn, and the next full breath cycle.
- You may notice from time to time that your attention is pulled away by a distraction, whether thought, sound, emotion, whatever it happens to be. This is not a problem; it is the nature of the human mind. There are two ways in which you can work with distraction:

- ❏ Gently and kindly bring your attention back to the breath, over and over again. This is the practice of cultivating the ability to attend; or
- ❏ Release your attention from the breath and let your attention focus on the distraction of thought, sound, or emotion. Notice that the thoughts or other distractions come and go and change in quality. Try to avoid creating a story around the distraction or adding a "thought to the thought." Just notice what is there and the changing quality of the distraction. When that distraction no longer holds your attention, bring your focus back to your anchor, to your breath.
- If thoughts become repetitive or intrusive, you may wish to try adding a mental note, such as "thinking" or "worrying" or "planning." By adding these mental notes, one is better able to stay present in the meditation; it helps to observe patterns in your experience objectively and to avoid getting caught up in emotional reactions.
- Simply observe what is predominant in the mind and in the body and be present and accepting of what is.
- When you find your attention is pulling away, bring it back to the breath. This is the practice, training the mind to be present and strengthening the "mindfulness muscle." The more you practice, the easier it becomes to notice when you are distracted and the easier it is to maintain attention.
- Let us close this meditation by wishing ourselves well. You may repeat these words or whatever words call to you: "May I be safe and protected. May I be happy and healthy. May I live my life with joy and ease. May I be peaceful."

A 2010 study, conducted at Harvard University and distributed through a smartphone app, utilized data collected from 2,250 people living in the U.S. Study results indicated that the frequency of individuals thinking about what is and is not happening occurs at nearly the same rate, and that individuals are more unhappy during times of mind wandering than experiencing the present moment (Killingsworth & Gilbert, 2010). Thus, the researchers concluded that "A human mind is a wandering mind and a wandering mind is an unhappy mind. The ability to think about what is not happening is a cognitive achievement that comes at an emotional cost." (Killingsworth & Gilbert, 2010, p. 932).

Through mindfulness practices, we learn the ability to "tame the mind," and by doing so, we are also able to relax the body. Similar to training the physical body in preparation for a race, we can strengthen the "mindfulness muscle" by redirecting the wandering mind back to the breath over and over again, cultivating the ability to attend to the present and find wisdom and tranquility.

Starting a Meditation Practice

Learning how to work with the breathing patterns or focusing on another neutral object as the anchor for one's attention is the foundational exercise for starting a mindfulness practice. Many, if not all, of us have a very difficult time turning off our thoughts. As indicated earlier, the wandering mind is our default mode: cultivating the ability to attend and focus takes strong intentions and regular practice. It is important to set aside time for daily practice. In the busyness of life, it can be difficult to find time to practice; moreover, one may believe that this act of "non-doing" is in conflict with goal orientation and perpetuates living life as human doings instead of human beings. Practicing mindfulness in the morning, before the onslaught of the busy day, is typically ideal since our minds tend to be quieter in the early day, allowing us to start our day instead of our day starting us.

Mindfulness is about putting yourself first, knowing that investing in your own health and well-being is critical to sustaining the capacity to care for others. We cannot give and do for others if we are not first caring for ourselves. Treat this as an investment in your own health and well-being, the gift of self-care. Ongoing research indicates that mindfulness practice is as essential, if not more essential, than physical fitness in preventing illness and disease and living a high quality life (Greater Good, 2014).

While mindfulness practice is beautifully simple and completely accessible to all, it can be very difficult to achieve due to the strength of the habitually wandering and distracted mind. We in the healthcare profession, spend an inordinate amount of time thinking and, as a result, often lose connection with our physical bodies. Thus, mindfulness practice helps to overcome that disjunction and develop mind–body connections. The goal is to incorporate up to 20 minutes or more of daily meditation practice. The practices can be spread throughout the day, if more convenient.

STOP: Moving Out of Autopilot

The STOP practice is effective in creating space to step away from the worried and busy mind into the present moment. When we are fully present, we have access to the full range of options and resources available to us as responses to a given situation, which enables us to make better choices, feel better, and achieve better results. The practice, which goes by the acronym STOP, has four steps:

- **S** – Stop what you are doing; intentionally pause
- **T** – Take a breath
- **O** – Observe your thoughts, feelings, and emotions. Labeling them can have a calming effect and help to create spaciousness.
- **P** – Proceed with something that will support you in the moment; choose what is most important to you right now and go with it.

Relational Mindfulness

Mindfulness has the potential to deeply enhance our relationships by improving the power of our presence and strengthening our ability to relate and connect deeply with others. Such attunement allows you to focus your mind and attention on the internal world of another, which sparks the sense of truly being "felt" by another person (Siegel, 2007). Through being present with those in our lives, whether our friends and family, professional colleagues, or patients and their families, we have the possibility to repair relationships, transform connections, reduce suffering, and heal.

Bringing Mindfulness into the Workplace

There are a number of ways in which nurses can lead efforts to bring mindfulness into their organizations and into their practices of caring for patients and families. The time for change is now, and mindfulness is precisely the agent that is needed to transform patient care, heal the healers, and cultivate work environments where healthcare workers can be their best to give their best.

The Path to Mindfulness

Think of mindfulness as another helpful tool that you can use to break out of the habits of autopilot and reactivity. While the practice is actually quite simple, it requires discipline and intentionality to cultivate a new way of being versus doing. Mindfulness teaches us how to separate ourselves from ongoing and current train of thinking and instead stand aside as an objective observer; this allows us to cultivate a stance of objectivity and disidentification; that is, to distance yourself from any particular self-presentation. Learning how to connect more closely to the sensations of the body than to the thought narratives that we tell ourselves permits a sense of calm, clarity, and concentration. Such acuity allows us to break the pattern of reactivity and instead access our full repertoire of resources and higher quality thinking. By doing so, we find spaciousness, relaxation, and ease.

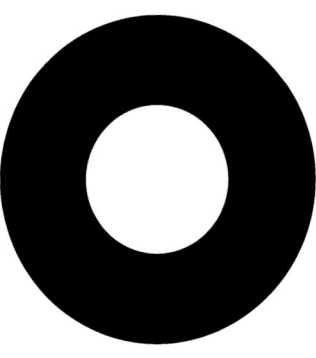
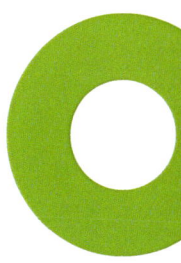

A Guide for Your Mindfulness Journey

- **Begin your own mindfulness practice.** You cannot talk about its transformative powers if you do not experience it yourself. Your own practice will further develop you as a leader.
- **Deeply understand the science.** There is no shortage of books and published articles on mindfulness. Become very curious about the practice and the science so that you are comfortable explaining the potential benefits.
- **Go where the water is already flowing.** Explore whether any other efforts are already underway in your organization to which mindfulness can be synergistic. For example, are there culture transformation initiatives underway that mindfulness can potentiate? Where else can you "attach?"
- **Build the business case.** Portray the potential benefits of a mindfulness initiative, including improved health and patient care, financial profitability, and reduced underlying costs, in terms that your leadership understands and values.
- **Expect resistance.** Despite appearing increasingly mainstream, mindfulness is still not well understood by the masses. Build consensus with other key stakeholders.
- **Recruit a strong executive sponsor.** This is critical to removing roadblocks, ensuring access to resources, and dealing with detractors.
- **Begin with a pilot.** Start small, and plan to collect data to address key questions that are important to your organization. There are several free survey instruments available in the public domain that have been used extensively for mindfulness research.
- **Engage a certified mindfulness facilitator to deliver the program.** Skillful and ethical teachers have many years of personal meditation practice and extensive experience working with people from a variety of backgrounds.
- **Measure and communicate impact.** This is critical to raising the visibility of your efforts and gaining buy-in for expansion to larger populations. Be mindful of the need for institutional review board approval for any research involving human subjects. Plan to publish findings outside of your organization.
- **Speak about your experience.** Share your learning and insights so that others may also benefit. The more we do so, with integrity and compassion, the more we can continue to address the real needs of people in pain and suffering.

References

Aiken, L.H., Clarke, S.P., Sloane, D.M., Sochalski, J., & Silber, J.H. (2002). Hospital nurse staffing and patient mortality, nurse burnout, and job dissatisfaction. *The Journal of the American Medical Association, 288*(16), 1987–1993.

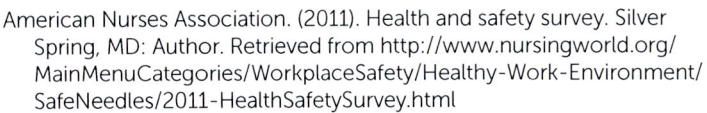

American Nurses Association. (2011). Health and safety survey. Silver Spring, MD: Author. Retrieved from http://www.nursingworld.org/MainMenuCategories/WorkplaceSafety/Healthy-Work-Environment/SafeNeedles/2011-HealthSafetySurvey.html

America's Health Insurance Plans. (2013). *Comprehensive assessment of ACA factors that will affect individual market premiums in 2014*. Washington, DC: Author. Retrieved from http://www.ahip.org/MillimanReportACA2013/

Baron, J. (2007). *Thinking and deciding* (4th ed.). New York, NY: Cambridge University Press.

Bazarko, D., Cate, R., Azocar, F., & Kreitzer, MJ. (2013). The impact of an innovative mindfulness-based stress reduction program on the health and well-being of nurses employed in a corporate setting. *Journal of Workplace Behavioral Health, 28*(2), 107–133.

Benson, H. (1975). *The relaxation response*. New York, NY: William Morrow and Company, Inc.

Brown, K.W., & Ryan, R.M. (2003). The benefits of being present: Mindfulness and its role in psychological well-being. *Journal of Personality and Social Psychology, 84*(4), 22–848.

Buerhaus, P., Donelan, K., Ulrich, B., Norman, L., & Dittus, R. (2006). State of the registered nurse workforce in the United States. *Nursing Economic$, 24*, 6–13.

Croskerry, P. (2003). The importance of cognitive errors in diagnosis and strategies to minimize them. *Academic Medicine, 78*(8), 775–780.

Davidson, R., Kabat-Zinn, J., Schumacher, J., Rosenkranz, M., Muller, D., Santorelli, S., & Sheridan, J. (2003). Alterations in brain and immune function produced by mindfulness meditation. *Psychosomatic Medicine, 65*(4), 564–570.

Elfering, A., Semmer, N.K., & Grebner, S. (2006). Work stress and patient safety: Observer-rated work stressors as predictors of characteristics of safety-related events reported by young nurses. *Ergonomics, 49*(5–6), 457–469. DOI: 10.1080/00140130600568451

Epel, E., Puterman, E., Lin, J., Blackburn, E., Lazaro, A., & Mendes, W. (2013). Wandering minds and aging cells. *Clinical Psychological Science, 1,* 75–83.

Gilboa, S., Shirom, A., Fried, Y., & Cooper, C. (2008). A meta-analysis of work demand stressors and job performance: Examining main and moderating effects. *Personnel Psychology, 61,* 227–272.

Greater Good: The science of a meaningful life. (2014). What is mindfulness? Berkeley, CA: Author. Retrieved from http://greatergood.berkeley.edu/topic/mindfulness/definition

Greeson, J.M. (2009). Mindfulness research update 2008. *Complementary Health Practice Review, 14*, 10–18.

Grossman, P., Niemann, L., Schmidt, S., & Walach, H. (2004). Mindfulness-based stress reduction and health benefits: A meta-analysis. *Journal of Psychosomatic Research, 57*, 35–43.

Hart, P. (2013). *Mind–body therapies*. Minneapolis, MN: University of Minnesota Center for Spirituality & Healing and Charleson Meadows. Retrieved from http://www.takingcharge.csh.umn.edu/explore-healing-practices/what-are-mind-body-therapies

Hölzel, B., Carmody, J., Vangel, M., Congleton, C., Yerramsetti, S., Gard, T., & Lazar, S. (2011). Mindfulness practice leads to increases in regional brain gray matter density. *Psychiatry Research: Neuroimaging, 191*(1), 36–43.

Jha A., Stanley E., Kiyonaga, A., Wong, L., & Gelfand, L., (2010). Examining the protective effects of mindfulness training on working memory capacity and affective experience. *Emotion, 10*(1), 54–64. DOI: 10.1037/a0018438

Jennings, B. (2008). Work stress and burnout among nurses: Role of the work environment and working conditions. In R.G. Hughes (Ed.), *Patient safety and quality: An evidence-based handbook for nurses* (pp. 137–158). AHRQ Publication No. 08-0043. Rockville, MD: Agency for Healthcare Research and Quality. Retrieved from http://www.ahrq.gov/qual/nurseshdbk/nurseshdbk.pdf

Kabat-Zinn, J. (2009). *Full catastrophe living: Using the wisdom of your body and mind to face stress, pain, and illness.* New York, NY: Bantam Dell.

Killingsworth, M., & Gilbert, D. (2010). A wandering mind is an unhappy mind. *Science, 330*, 932.

Krasner, M., Epstein, R., Beckman, H., Suchman, A., Chapman, B., Mooney, C., & Quill, T. (2009). Association of an educational program in mindful communication with burnout, empathy, and attitudes among primary care physicians. *Journal of the American Medical Association, 302*, 1284–1293.

Lin, J., Epel, E., & Blackburn, E. (2011). Telomeres and lifestyle factors: Roles in cellular aging. *Mutation Research, 73*(1–2), 85–89.

McCarney, R., Schulz, J., & Grey, R. (2012). Effectiveness of mindfulness-based interventions in reducing symptoms of depression: A meta-analysis. *European Journal of Psychotherapy & Counseling, 14*(3), 279–299.

Mrazek, M., Franklin, M., Phillips, D., Baird, B., & Schooler, J. (2013). Mindfulness training improves working memory capacity and GRE performance while reducing mind wandering. *Psychological Science, 24*(5), 776–781. DOI: 10.1177/0956797612459659

O'Conner, T., O'Halloran, D., & Shanahan, F. (2000). The stress response and the hypothalamic-pituitary-adrenal axis: From molecule to melancholia. *QJM: An International Journal of Medicine, 93*(6), 323–333. DOI:10.1093/qjmed/93.6.323

Rosenberg, E. (2013). Meditation and emotion. In A. Fraser (Ed.), *The healing power of meditation* (pp. 66–78). Boston, MA: Shambhala Publications, Inc.

Sansoucie, D., Steckel, A., Messina, B., Greenfield, J., Kealey, C., Bratby, K., & Boughton, S. (2005). The relationship between serenity and burnout among nurses. Paper presented at the Sigma Theta Tau International Nursing Research Congress, November 14, 2005, Indianapolis, IN.

Sibinga, E., & Wu, A., (2010). Clinician mindfulness and patient safety. *Journal of the American Medical Association, 304*(22), 3532–3533.

Siegel, D. (2007). *The mindful brain*. New York, NY: W.W. Norton & Company, Inc.

Shapiro, S.L., Astin, J.A., Bishop, S., & Cordova, M. (2005). Mindfulness-based stress reduction for health care professionals: Results from a randomized trial. *International Journal of Stress Management, 12*, 164–176.

Shapiro, S.L., Carlson, L.E., Astin, J.A., & Freedman, B. (2006). Mechanisms of mindfulness. *Journal of Clinical Psychology, 62*(3), 373–386.

Smalley, S., & Winston, D. (2010). *Fully present: The science, art and practice of mindfulness*. Philadelphia, PA: Da Capo Press.

Zangaro, G., & Soeken, K. (2007). A meta-analysis of studies of nurses' job satisfaction. *Research in Nursing & Health, 30*(4), 445–458.

Zeidan, F., Martucci, K., Kraft, R., McHaffie, J., & Coghill, R. (2013). Neural correlates of mindfulness meditation-related anxiety relief. *Social Cognitive and Affective Neuroscience, 31*(14), 5540–5548. DOI:10.1093/scan/nst041

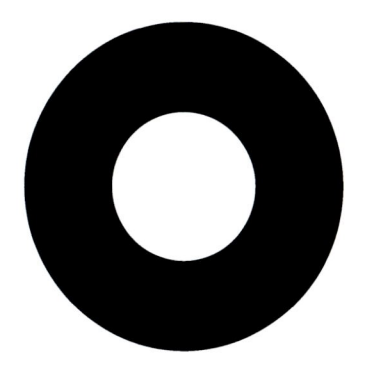

Suggested Readings and Resources

American Nurses Association (2014). HealthyNurse™. Retrieved from http://www.anahealthynurse.org.

Fraser, A. (2013). *The healing power of meditation. Leading experts on Buddhism, psychology, and medicine explore the health benefits of contemplative practice.* Boston, MA: Shambhala Publications.

Goleman, D. (2013). *Focus: The hidden driver of excellence.* New York, NY: HarperCollins.

Greater Good: *The science of a meaningful life: A video series.* (2014). Featured mindfulness stories. Berkeley, CA: Author. Retrieved from http://greatergood.berkeley.edu/topic/mindfulness

Kabat-Zinn, J. (2009). *Full catastrophe living: Using the wisdom of your body and mind to face stress, pain, and illness.* New York, NY: Bantam Dell.

Spotlight Six Software, LLC. Insight Meditation Timer. Retrieved from https://insighttimer.com/

Siegel, D. (2010). *Mindsight: The science of personal transformation.* New York, NY: Bantam Books.

Smalley, S., & Winston, D. (2010). *Fully present: The science, art and practice of mindfulness*. Philadelphia, PA: Da Capo Press.

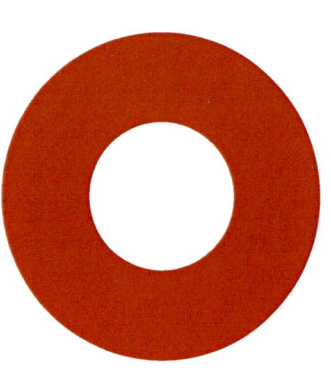

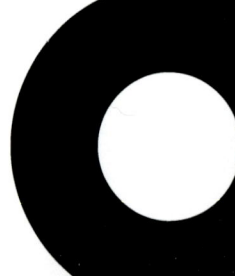